Alkali

Drastically Impro........Areas of Your Health, Feel Energized and Start Losing Weight!

By Elena Garcia and James Adler

www.HolisticWellnessBooks.com

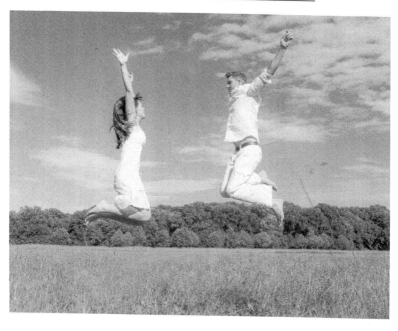

recording or otherwise, without the prior written permission of the author and the publishers.

The book is not intended to provide medical advice or to take the place of medical advice and treatment from your personal physician. Readers are advised to consult their own doctors or other qualified health professionals regarding the treatment of medical conditions. The authors shall not be held liable or responsible for any misunderstanding or misuse of the information contained in this book. The information is not intended to diagnose, treat or cure any disease.

It is important to remember that the authors of this book are not a doctor/ medical professional. Only opinions based upon their own personal experiences or research are cited. THE AUTHORS DO NOT OFFER MEDICAL ADVICE or prescribe any treatments. For any health or medical issues – you should be talking to your doctor first.

Table of Contents

Introduction

Thank you for taking an interest in our book, it really means a lot to us!

This book is designed to give you a comprehensive overview of the Alkaline Diet. It explains exactly how to change your lifestyle so that you can think clearly, have unlimited amounts of energy, detoxify your system and lose weight!

We are Elena and James, a married couple, who together found the ultimate lifestyle. We wanted to create this book to enable you to embrace this diet and transition easily into a lifestyle that will literally change your life, as it has ours.

When we embarked on this journey we had no idea all of the benefits we would reap. We were able to burn fat more efficiently, had a huge increase in our mental focus and creativity. Energy is now abundant and we feel amazing.

The alkaline way is the only way to live for us now. It is a life-altering experience for any who dedicate themselves to it. The alkaline lifestyle is a body and mind diet; a truly holistic perspective. We have never felt better, and we hope that you will join us.

Thanks again for downloading our book, we hope you enjoy it!

Elena & James

Welcome Gift+Wellness Newsletter
Free Complimentary eBook

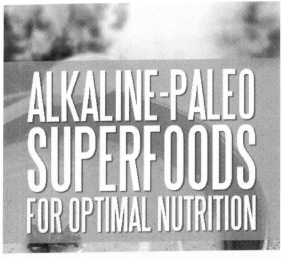

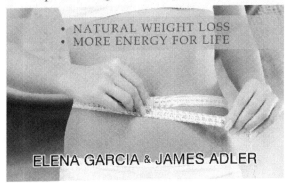

Download link:

Go to: www.bitly.com/alkapaleofree

Problems with your download?

Contact us: elenajamesbooks@gmail.com

Chapter 1 Alkaline Lifestyle for Holistic Health

We, as a couple, adore Tony Robbins. He is motivated, positive and his energy is infectious. We have learned so much from him. Alkalinity is no different. We heard him speak of "going green" and our lives have been transformed forever. Most people hear the term "going green" and think of recycling or doing other things in regard to the environment. We were under the same impression. After listening to a seminar on Tony's enthusiasm for alkalinity and his breakdown of its life changing benefits, we were enthralled. He has not only put us on the road to positive thinking and personal success, he has shown us that living an alkaline lifestyle will only propel and enhance all of the other ideas and tools for success he has given us. It is another way that shows us how to attain OVERALL health and wellness. When the body is able to function at one hundred percent, so is the mind.

Going green is a way to describe an alkaline lifestyle because the focus is on green vegetables in general, as they are the most alkaline food you can ingest. By ingesting alkaline foods and beverages (he is a big advocate of alkaline water and nutritious green smoothies which we now embrace as well) you can alkalize your entire system, causing it to function at its best. The benefits of the alkaline diet are numerous. Let us name a few:

WEIGHT LOSS

An alkaline diet will assist you in losing weight. One way that it does this is obvious. All of the foods you will be eating are very healthy, rich in minerals and low calorie in general.

You will also be reducing the amount of acid in your body. The body stores fat in order to protect itself from an abundance of acid. It is a self-preservation method. This is part of the reason why people who exercise a lot and drink an excess of caffeine cannot seem to lose those extra pounds. Their bodies are clinging to that fat to minimize the effects of all of the acid in their systems. Caffeine is really acid-forming and it's not the most sustainable source of energy.

Another benefit of an alkaline lifestyle in regard to weight loss is that alkaline systems have more oxygen in their cells. Oxygen is a very essential part of eliminating fat cells from the body. The more oxygen in your system, the more efficient your metabolism will be. James learned this as he had previously believed that just because he was getting older, his metabolism was slowing down. He was able to speed it back up by eating alkaline, burning off more fat than ever before!

ENERGY

Now James is normally a pretty energized person. He can wake right up and get started with his day. He was never even too interested in caffeine. I (Elena), on the other hand, felt pretty lethargic and listless on a regular basis. Caffeine was my buddy. I am half-Spanish and half-Italian and drinking coffee is deeply rooted in my culture. I started drinking coffee when I was only eleven! Everyone drinks coffee in Italy, where I grew up. People socialize drinking coffee in the streets. Everyone is always up for a cappuccino or espresso! Most of the Italians would even tell you that coffee is super healthy! While I do agree that having a nice cup of coffee is great as a treat, we should not depend on it for energy. Moderation is the key.

Well, thanks to my new alkaline lifestyle I have totally changed my attitude and managed to control my caffeine addiction. I was one of those people who did not even want to converse until I had downed my first cup of coffee. I thought that I was simply hormonal or sleep deprived. I always envied other people who had a constant supply of energy (James thought Tony Robbins was just naturally hyper). Little did we know that an alkaline lifestyle could provide that for us!

Going green does not only give you energy for the obvious reason that you are eating many more healthy, energizing vitamins. You are negating the acid induced lethargy that is brought on by an unhealthy acid-forming diet.

Not only do our bodies need an abundance of oxygen to lose weight, we need oxygen in our cells to energize us. The lack of oxygen in our cells causes fatigue. No, it is not just because you worked too late or partied to hard the night before. It is internal. If your cells are trying to function in a highly acidic environment they will not be able to transfer oxygen in an efficient manner; leading of course to exhaustion.

Cells in the body also make something that is called adenosine triphosphate (ATP). If your system is very acidic, it has an adverse effect on the ability of your cells to produce it. In the scientific world it is known as the "energy current of life." The ATP molecule contains the energy that we need to accomplish most things that we do (both internally and externally).

BODILY FUNCTIONS

Another benefit of the alkaline lifestyle is that your body will be able to function at an optimum level instead of being inhibited by acids:

- Your heart beat is thrown off by acidic wastes in the body. The stomach suffers greatly from over-acidity.

- The liver's job is to get rid of acid toxins, but also to produce alkaline enzymes. By simply reducing your acid intake you can internally boost your alkalinity thanks to your liver!

- Your pancreas thrives on alkalinity. Too much acid in your system throws off your pancreas. If you eat alkaline foods, your pancreas is able to regulate your blood sugars.

- Your kidneys also help to keep your body alkaline. When they are overwhelmed by an acidic diet they cannot do their job (and no one wants a kidney stone-just ask James!-OUCH).

- The lymph fluids function most efficiently in an alkaline system. They remove acid waste. Acidic systems not only have a slower lymph flow causing acids to be stored; they can also cause acids to be reabsorbed through lymphatic ducts in your intestines that would normally be excreted.

MENTAL FOCUS

Tony Robbins is the master of his mind. He knows how to use it to fuel his decisions and emotions. He enlightened us to the fact that alkalinity of the system is one of the best ways to focus and strengthen the mind. Just as the rest of the body is poorly effected by acid-forming foods and other toxins, so is your brain. And as we all know, it should be possible to control your emotions and decision making with your mind. Guess what? If your body is too acidic and is not alkaline, your mental clarity will be cloudy, your decision making could be off, as well as your emotional state.

DETOX

Another huge benefit of an alkaline lifestyle is detoxification. First, you are going to be cutting out foods that are constantly adding toxins to your system. Secondly, you are going to be eating foods that allow your body to detox and rid itself of the acids that have built up in your system all this time. When we detoxify our bodies, our emotions, bodily functions and mental functions are able operate at their optimum levels.

The amount of benefits that come with living alkaline are numerous. As you help your body rebalance its optimal blood pH you will find, as we did, that you have never felt better. We are still seeing improvement and reaping the rewards of this holistic approach to not only eating alkaline foods, but living alkaline.

Chapter 2 Going Alkaline in an Easy Way

Alkaline vs. Acidic? Sounds like the title fight for a light weight boxing match. In reality it is a fight, a fight for the pH balance of your body. pH levels are basically the measure of how acidic a liquid is. Our bodies function optimally when our blood is at about 7.35 ph. pH levels range from 0 to 14. 0 is the highest level of acidity, but basically everything 0-7 would be considered acidic. The 7-14 range is alkaline.

Before we dive into complicated pH discussions, here is one thing to understand:

-The alkaline <u>diet is not about changing or "raising" your pH</u>. This is where many alkaline guides go wrong. You see, our body is smart enough to self-regulate our pH for us, no matter what we eat. Unfortunately, when you constantly bombard your body with acid-forming foods (for example processed foods, fast food, alcohol, sugar, and even too much meat) you torture your body with an incredible stress. Why? Well because it has to work harder to maintain that optimal pH...

Here's simple example...

Imagine you immerse yourself in a bath filled with ice. You say, but hey, my body can self-regulate its optimal temperature, right? And yes, it can. But it will eventually collapse and you will get ill. The same happens with nutrition and our blood pH. You can spend years indulging in toxic, processed, acid-forming foods that only deprive your body of its vital nutrients, saying: "But hey, my body will self-regulate its optimal blood pH".

And again, it will...but sooner or later it will give up and manifest a disease. It will accumulate fat as its natural defense function to protect your body from over-acidity. We don't wanna end up there, right?

So, to sum up- the alkaline diet is a natural, holistic system, a nutritional lifestyle that advocates consumption of fresh, unprocessed foods that are rich in nutrients. These are called alkaline foods and they help your body stimulate its optimal healing functions. Yes! A healthy body needs nutrients and fresh fruits and vegetables are great for that.

The problem is that nowadays, most diets are filled with acid-forming foods that eventually make it hard for the body to regulate its optimal, healthy blood pH and artificial sweeteners do the same. Acidosis is very common in this day and age thanks to things we drink as well: coffee, alcohol, and sodas all have an acidic effect on our bodies. Not to mention the chemicals many people take in through things like smoking and drugs (even prescription drugs have this effect).

There are many ways that you could become acidic. Eating acid forming foods, stress, taking in too many toxins, and bodily processes all cause acidity in the body. Our internal systems try to balance themselves out and bring pH up with the help of alkaline minerals that we can ingest through our diet. If we do not take in a higher percentage of alkaline than acidic foods, we can become too acidic.

When you are acidic, it makes every process that your body normally does much more difficult or impossible for it to accomplish. We cannot absorb the beneficial nutrients we need from our food properly. Our cells are not able to produce energy efficiently. Our bodies are not able to fix damaged cells properly. We will not be able to detoxify properly. Fatigue and illness will drag you down. Sounds horrible; does it not? Here are some signs that you are overly acidic. This list was eye opening for the both of us, as we almost checked off the entire list between the two of us!

- ✓ Feeling tired all the time. You have no physical or mental drive at all.

- ✓ You always feel cold. (This was a big one for me, Elena)

- ✓ You get sick easily.

- ✓ You are depressed or just feel "blah" all the time for no real reason (I, Elena, had this problem and thought it was hormonal changes).

- ✓ You are easily overstimulated and stressed by noise, light, etc. (I, James, could never figure out why I was like this).

- ✓ You get headaches for no apparent reason (This fit me, Elena, to a tee).

- ✓ You get watery eyes or inflamed eyelids.

- ✓ Your teeth are sensitive and may crack or chip (I, Elena, always fought this).

- ✓ Your gums are inflamed and you are susceptible to canker sores (I, James, thought this was genetic, but now know better).

- ✓ You have recurring bouts with throat problems including tonsillitis (both of us).

- ✓ Acidic stomach with acid indigestion and reflux is always an issue (James hated this).

- ✓ Your fingernails crack, split, and break (I, Elena, battled this with nasty acrylic nails because mine would never grow).

- ✓ You have super dry hair that sheds and is hay-like with split ends (Elena, again).

- ✓ You have dry, ashy skin (both of us!)

- ✓ Your skin breaks out in acne or is irritated when you sweat (both of us had this problem).

- ✓ You get leg cramps and spasms (this includes restless leg syndrome which they told James he had).

Of course remember that whenever you experience any health/medical conditions you need to see your doctor first and get a checkup.

Changing your diet to one that is full of alkaline foods is one of the easiest and best things you can do for your overall health. We were so ecstatic that we did! If you are acidic, as we were, you should change your diet immediately. You should aim to intake 80 percent alkaline-forming foods and the remaining 20 percent can be acid-forming foods (for example some animal products). Fast food and junk food should be ditched forever! You don't need it. Once your pH diet is back on track, you can shift as we did to a 60 percent alkaline and 40 percent acid to maintain a high pH. Although, if you CAN stick to 80/20 then why not? We aim to eat this way most of the time.

Many people complain that this diet is hard to follow.

But the way we see it is this- it's perfect! Plus it's not a diet, it's a lifestyle.

What we really like about it, is that you don't have to be 100% perfect. It's enough to be 80% awesome and 20% relaxed. You can even swap the 80/20 rule for 70/30 rule meaning that about 70% of your diet should be fresh, nutrient dense alkaline-forming foods and the remaining 30% can be acid-forming foods (however they still should be fresh and organic, for example grass-fed meat or organic eggs, some gluten-free grains and legumes).

Many alkaline diet and lifestyle lovers decide to go vegan and we very often get asked by our readers:

In order to get alkaline, do I have to go vegan?

We believe it's totally up to you. Alkaline diet is pretty vegan in its design, and alkaline and vegan concepts very often overlap. However, you don't have to go 100% vegan to be alkaline (unless you want to).

You see people choose a vegan lifestyle for other personal and spiritual reasons- like love for the planet, love for the animals and other. And yes, many people go alkaline and use it as a starting point to eventually go fully vegan.

Again, the decision is totally up to you. This is not a book on veganism, we are not here to preach to you, and we just want to give you more than enough of information, inspiration and motivation so that you create your own way, something that works for you.

What many alkaline diet followers do to begin with is to create a strong, plant-based foundation for their diet and then add small amounts of fish. Many alkaline diet gurus, including its pioneer Doctor Robert O'Young include fish and fish oils in their diet and recommendations.

The most important thing is to do what works for you. All you need to keep in mind is to aim to eat 70-80% alkaline and try to eat more vegan/plant-based, even if you are not fully vegan.

The recipe section will give you some ideas!

For the most part, as a general rule, green veggies, many fruits, lentils, and seeds/nuts are considered alkaline. While animals, their byproducts, and all grains and legumes are acidic in general.

What are alkaline foods? Is it about their pH?

No, luckily it's much, much easier. We don't care about the food's pH in its natural form...All we care about is the effect that the food has on the body after it has been consumed and metabolized. For example, lemons, grapefruits and limes are considered alkaline-forming foods.

What? Elena? James! Are you out of your mind? Everyone knows lemons are acidic...

Well, let us repeat again. Lemons are acidic as far as their taste and ph. in their natural state are concerned. But, they are full of alkaline minerals and low in sugar which makes them alkaline-forming foods.

At the same time, oranges contain more sugar which makes them less alkaline-forming.

Let us repeat:

Some charts determine acidity or alkalinity of the food before it is consumed & others (like the ones we follow and recommend) are more interested in the effect the food has on the body after it has been consumed.

It's really that simple!

As a general rule, alkaline foods are:
-rich in minerals and vitamins
-fresh, not packaged
-not fermented

-low in sugar (all kinds of sugar are acid-forming)

-plant-based

-mostly raw or slightly cooked

-caffeine-free

-chemical-free

-provide hydration

As a general rule, acid-forming foods are:

-full of chemicals

-low in nutrients

-high in sugar

-contain caffeine, alcohol, toxins

-processed

-packaged

-fermented

-contain artificial ingredients

-animal byproducts

So let's have a look at the food lists. We think that after our intro it will be easier for you to understand the difference between alkaline and acid forming foods, even without looking at the charts...

One more thing- we base our food lists on Doctor Young's latest research.

We know it is quite confusing to see so many different charts online. We have been there.

The reason why so many other charts show such disparity is because they base their classifications on the readings for the so called PRAL which stands for Potential Renal Acid Load research. Unfortunately, this is not a reliable source of practical information for us.

Why?

Well PRAL tests burn the food at an extreme temperature and then take a read of the 'ash' that is left behind and what it's pH is.

While this will give a read of its alkalinity from the mineral content of the food, by burning it at such a high temperature they also burn away sugar. And sugar is very acid-forming...

That is why on some charts high sugar fruits are listed as super alkaline. Now we are not saying that fruits are bad for you, most fruits are neutral or mildly acid forming and great as a natural snack or a part of a balanced diet. But they are not as alkalizing as most veggies are.

Some charts determine acidity or alkalinity on the food before it is consumed & others like the ones we list below, are more interested in the effect the food has on the body after it has been consumed.

ALKALIZING VEGETABLES

Asparagus

Broccoli

Chili

Pepper

Zucchini

Dandelion

Snowpeas

Green Beans

String Beans

Runner Beans

Spinach

Kale

Wakame

Kelp

Collards

Chives

Endive

Chard

Cabbage

Sweet Potato

Mint

Ginger

Coriander

Basil

Brussels Sprouts

Cauliflower

Carrot

Beetroot

Eggplant

Garlic

Onion

Parsley

Celery

Cucumber

Watercress

Lettuce

Peas

Broad Beans

New Potato

Pumpkin

Radish

ALKALIZING FRUITS

Avocado

Tomato

Lemon

Lime

Grapefruit

Fresh Coconut

Pomegranate

ALKALIZING PROTEIN

Almonds,

Chestnuts,

Millet,

Protein Powders (we love hemp)

ALKALINE OILS

Avocado Oil

Coconut Oil

Flax Oil

Udo's Oil

Olive Oil

Other:

Alkaline Water

GMO-free Tofu (neutral)

Fresh Goat & Almond Milk

Herbal Tea

Buckwheat Pasta

ALKALINE SUPERFOODS:

Wheatgrass

Barley Grass

Kamut Grass

Dog Grass

Shave Grass

Oat Grass

Soy Sprouts

Alfalfa Sprouts

Amaranth Sprouts

Broccoli Sprouts

Fenugreek Sprouts

Kamut Sprouts

Mung Bean Sprouts

Quinoa Sprouts

Radish Sprouts

Spelt Sprouts

ALKALINE-FRIENDLY BREADS:

Sprouted Bread

Sprouted Wraps

Gluten/Yeast-Free Breads & Wraps

ALKALIZING SWEETENERS
-Stevia (natural)

ALKALIZING SPICES & SEASONINGS
-Chili Peppers,

-Cinnamon,

-Curry,

-Ginger,

-Herbs,

-Sea Salt,

ALKALIZING NUTS AND SEEDS
Almonds

Coconut

Flax Seeds

Pumpkin Seeds

Sesame Seeds

Sunflower Seeds

ACID SWEETENERS
Carob, Corn Syrup, Sugar

ACID BEVERAGES

Alcohol, Coffee, Soda

ACID TOXINS AND DRUGS
All drugs, Weed killers, Insecticides, Tobacco

ACID MEAT:
Bacon

Beef

Clams

Corned Beef

Eggs

Lamb

Lobster

Mussels

Organ Meats

Venison

Fish

Oyster

Pork

Rabbit

Sausage

Scallops

Shellfish

Shrimp

Tuna

Turkey

Veal

MIDLY ACID-FORMING/NEUTRAL FRUITS:

Apple

Apricot

Dates

Grapes

Mango

Peach

Pear

Prunes

Raisins

Raspberries

Strawberries

Tropical Fruits

Cantaloupe

Cranberries

Currants

Honeydew Melon

Orange

Pineapple

Plum

ACID FORMING DAIRY AND EGGS

Butter

Cheese

Milk

Whey

Yogurt

Cottage Cheese

Ice Cream

Sour Cream

Soy Cheese

Eggs

MIDLY ACID FORMING NUTS AND SEEDS

Cashews

Peanuts

Pecans

Pistachios

Walnuts

Brazil Nuts

Chestnuts

Hazelnuts

Macadamia Nuts

ACID FORMING OILS

Cooked Oil

Solid Oil (Margarine)

Oil Exposed to Heat,
Light or Air

ACID FORMING DRINKS

Alcohol

Black Tea

Coffee

Carbonated Water

Pasteurized Juice

Cocoa

Energy Drinks

Sports Drinks

Colas

Tap Water

Milk

Green Tea

Decaffeinated Drinks

Flavoured Water

ACID-FORMING SAUCES

Mayonnaise

Ketchup

Mustard

Soy Sauce

Pickles

Vinegar

Tabasco

Tamari

Wasabi

Other ACID-FORMING FOODS:

Mushrooms

Miso

White Breads, Pastas,

Rice & Noodles

Chocolate

Chips

Pizza

Biscuits

Cigarettes

Drugs

Candy!

Now, there is debate on quite a few things as to whether or not they are alkalizing or acidifying. Many charts lists them as neutral and this is what we believe make sense. The good thing about the alkaline lifestyle is that we do not have to eat 100 percent alkaline. As long as we are taking in MOSTLY alkalizing foods, we are still on track! Here are some of the debated foods:

-Apple Cider Vinegar
-Brazil Nuts,
-Brussels Sprouts,
-Buckwheat,
-Cashews,
-Chicken,
-Corn,
- Cottage Cheese,
-Eggs,
-Flax,
-Green Tea,
-Honey,
-Kombucha,
-Lima Beans,
-Potatoes,
-Pepitas,
-Quinoa,
-Sauerkraut,
-Soy,
-Squash,
-Sunflower Seeds,

-Tomatoes,

-Yogurt.

Use charts as a guide, but don't worry too much if you find it difficult to memorize or if you have doubts whether your favorite food is alkaline enough. I, Elena, keep one of my 'alkaline charts' in my wallet at all times to reference at the grocery store!

FREE COMPLIMENTARY
DOWNLOAD

We also have easy printable charts that you can download at no cost.

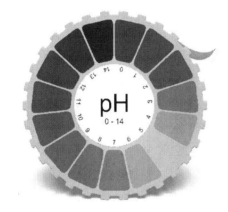

Download Link:

www.bitly.com/alkalinecharts

Problems with your download?

Email us at: elenajamesbooks@gmail.com

Chapter 3 Meal Plan and Recipes

Now, that you have a general idea on what is alkaline, what is acid, and what alkalinity can do for you; let us help you out with a meal plan and some recipes. Honestly, James is not a chef and if he can do it you can too! The great part about cooking for an alkaline diet is that you simply have to mix and match ingredients. Another bonus: you can eat as many raw components as you like! Cooking takes away from the alkalinity of many foods so if you like it raw, more power to you. If it is cooked, do not worry! It will still be alkaline!

We are big proponents of juicing. You can get so much raw alkaline nutrition from a glass. It is sometimes difficult to get as many raw green vegetables as you should in a day. Juicing is a great way to get concentrated alkaline nutrition. You can even save the pulp that most people toss away and use it in soups. It is full of fiber and alkaline nutrition!

Here is a three day meal plan to get you started. The recipes are included! Remember to use ORGANIC ingredients.

DAY ONE

Breakfast:

<u>Wake Up Smoothie</u>

- 1 Apple, green is best (take out the core)
- 4 Celery stalks
- 1 Cup baby Spinach
- 1 ripe Avocado
- 1 bunch cilantro (no stems)
- 3 cups spring water
- ½ fresh-squeezed lemon
- ¼ tsp cayenne pepper (optional)

1. Cut all into smaller pieces
2. Put water in blender
3. Blend and drink!

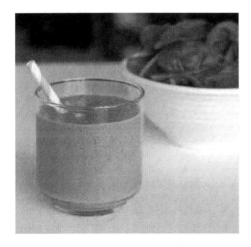

Lunch:

Cesar Kale Salad

- 1 bunch of Kale (torn)
- 1 cup raw sunflower seeds (shells removed of course)
- 1/3 cup raw almonds
- ¼ teaspoon cayenne
- ½ teaspoon paprika
- 2 minced garlic
- ¼ cup spring or filtered water
- 1 ½ teaspoon agave
- ½ teaspoon sea salt

1. Wash, dry and tear up kale
2. Put in a mixing bowl
3. Put all other ingredients in blender
4. Blend until smooth
5. Pour the mixture over the kale and mix well
6. Make sure all is coated and allow to marinate ten minutes
7. Plate and top with seeds
8. Enjoy!

Dinner:

Alkaline Stir-fry

- ½ of a squash (your choice) cut into 1 inch pieces
- 1 chopped onion
- 1 inch piece of ginger, chopped or grated
- 2 chopped cloves of garlic
- 2 cups chopped cabbage
- 2 cups spinach
- 1 chopped chili of your choice
- 2 tablespoons coconut oil
- ½ of a squeezed lemon (juice)
- Pinch of sea salt and pepper to your taste
- 1 tablespoon Braggs Aminos
- 2 tablespoons spring water

1. Heat coconut oil over medium heat in a big frying pan or wok
2. Fry up the onion for 3 minutes
3. Put in the ginger, chili, and garlic and cook for another minute stirring constantly
4. Add the squash, salt and pepper, keep cooking and stirring until squash is soft but not smooshy.
5. Add cabbage and spinach with the lemon juice and cook for 2 minutes

41

6. Remove from heat and toss in the Braggs

7. Enjoy!

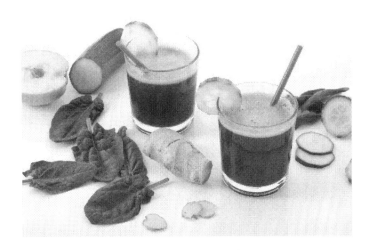

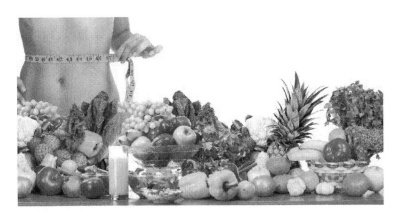

DAY TWO

Breakfast:

<u>Energy Juice</u>

- A cucumber
- 2 cups baby spinach
- 1 or 2 sticks of celery
- 1 cup chopped kale
- Juice of one lemon or lime

1. Juice and enjoy!

We love starting the day with a green juice or smoothie and a handful of raw almonds!

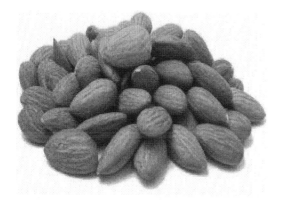

Lunch:

<u>**Cool Veggie Soup**</u>

- 1 avocado
- 1 zucchini
- 3 celery stalks
- 2 handfuls baby spinach
- ½ cup both parsley and cilantro
- ½ cup raw almonds
- Pinch of sea salt
- Pinch of cayenne
- 1 ½ cups of spring water (or 2 depending on how thick you want it)
- Juice of 1 lime

1. Cut any large ingredients into smaller pieces if necessary and put everything into a blender and mix well.
2. If you like you can warm it on the stove but I, James, love it cold.
3. Enjoy!

Dinner:

Veggie Soup

- 1 large onion (chopped)
- 3 garlic cloves (minced)
- 3 carrots (cut to your liking)
- 3 sweet potatoes (cubed)
- ½ squash (cubed)
- 2 tomatoes (diced)
- 4 celery stalks (chopped)
- 2 zucchini (chopped)
- 1 large bell pepper (seeded and chopped)
- 2 cups cooked millet
- Pinch sea salt
- 1/2 cup parsley (chopped) and 2 more tablespoons to garnish

Broth:

- ¼ both onion and cabbage
- 2 zucchini
- 4 of each: celery stalks and carrots
- ½ red bell pepper
- Filtered or spring water

1. For the broth, juice all the veggies.

2. Put onion and garlic in a pot with 2 tablespoons water.

3. Cook over medium until onion is clear.

4. Add the juice broth and 1 cup of water.

5. Heat to a simmer and then put in the carrots, sweet potatoes, and squash; simmer five minutes.

6. Throw in the zucchini and celery, cooking an additional five minutes.

7. Now, put in peppers, tomatoes, and cooked millet. Simmer five more minutes.

8. Season and add parsley.

9. Enjoy!

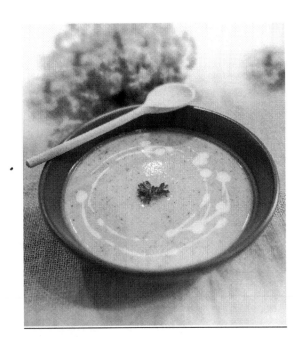

DAY THREE

Breakfast:
Spelt Pancakes

- 1 cup spelt flour
- 2 tablespoons baking powder
- Pinch sea salt
- 1 cup almond or hemp milk
- 1 tablespoon maple syrup
- 2 tablespoons sunflower oil (cold pressed)
- 1 ½ teaspoons pure vanilla
- Coconut oil to grease pan

1. Mix all dry ingredients in mixing bowl.
2. Mix all wet ingredients in a separate bowl.
3. Slowly add the wet mixture to the dry, stirring just until it is blended.
4. Let batter set for ten minutes.
5. Heat a large griddle or frying pan to medium and grease with coconut oil.
6. Pour batter onto pan, make size to your liking.
7. Cook for two minutes, or until little bubbles arise on top and sides.
8. When lightly browned on bottom flip and cook the same on the other side.

9. Serve and enjoy!

I, Elena, love mine with almond butter! You can use fruit, if you like, as a topping.

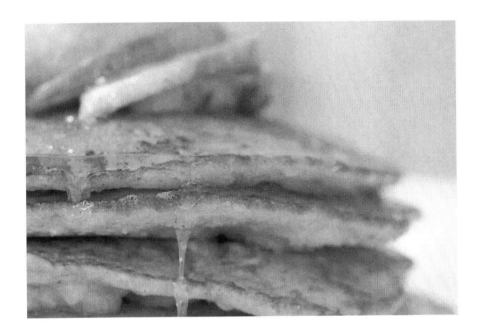

Lunch:

Alkaline Tabbouleh

- Juice of one lemon
- 1 c. Rinsed millet
- 2 c. Spring or filtered water
- 1 pinch sea salt
- 1/3 c. evoo (extra virigin olive oil)
- 2 cloves minced garlic
- 4 diced roma tomatoes
- 1 diced cucumber (English)
- ½ c. chopped green onion
- ¾ c. chopped parsley
- ¾ c. chopped mint

1. Boil water and add the rinsed millet. Simmer covered for about 20 minutes.
2. Cool for one hour.
3. Mix evoo, lemon juice, and garlic (set aside).
4. Put the vegetables in a large bowl and add cooled millet.
5. Add the dressing and stir well.
6. Season with sea salt and garnish with parsley and mint.

James likes this best after it has set for a few hours, but you can eat immediately!

Dinner:

Stuffed Spaghetti Squash

- 2 medium to large spaghetti squash
- 12 diced roma tomatoes
- 1 diced onion
- 4 cloves minced garlic
- 1.5 tablespoons evoo
- Sea salt to taste
- Pinch of stevia
- ¼ cup basil chopped
- 5 or 6 sundried tomatoes

1. Cut squash in half. Remove the seeds.
2. Place face down in pan with 2 cups of water.
3. Bake in oven at 300 degrees for an hour or until tender enough to pull out spaghetti strings.
4. While it is baking, fry up the onion and garlic in the evoo until onion is clear.
5. Put in the tomatoes (roma and sundried).
6. Turn heat to low and cook for 8 minutes.
7. Add half of the basil, salt and stevia (only a tad).
8. Take half of this mixture and blend in your blender.
9. After, put it back in with the other mixture.
10. Loosen the "noodles" in the squash.

11. Spoon sauce over the squash and sprinkle remaining basil.
12. Top with almond "cheese."

Almond "Cheese"

- 2/3 c. raw almonds
- 1 large clove garlic
- ¼ tsp sea salt

1. Put all ingredients in food processor or blender and mix until fine.

Chapter 4 How to Stay Motivated and On-track

As a couple who has successfully kept up our alkaline lifestyle for two years now, we can attest to the fact that the number one motivator in staying on track is how great you will feel. Every morning we wake up energized. We feel healthy because we are. We think clearly because we can. Why would we ever go back to feeling sick and lethargic?

There are some tips that we would like to share with you that can help to keep you going. This is my, Elena's, top tip: prepare snacks. Good snacks. Have them on hand or in the fridge at all times. Each time I go shopping I take the time to rinse my veggies and then cut them up, putting them in snack baggies or containers so that way I can grab and go! We also do the same with baggies of almonds (and other nuts of our preference) in the car.

Here are also some of the snack recipes that we use to stay on track:

Kale Chips

- Wash kale and rip the leaves off (I do about 5)

- Dry leaves

- Drizzle 1/2 tablespoon of coconut oil and some seasoning of your choice

- Mix it up all together in a mixing bowl or large baggie using your hand so that all the kale is oiled

- Lay them out on a baking sheet at 350 degrees for 10 minutes

While you're at it, place some kale through your juicer. Green juice is great for weight loss and mental focus.

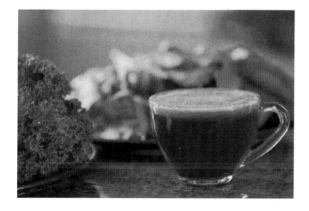

Hummus with Raw Veggies

- 1 can garbanzo beans drained

- 1 chopped zucchini

- 1 minced garlic clove

- About a handful each of fresh basil and parsley

- Salt and pepper to taste

- 4 tablespoons evoo (extra virigin olive oil)

- A big squeeze of lemon

Throw it all into a blender/food processor and enjoy with raw veggies!

ALKALINE WATER

Water is a key component in staying healthy in general, but is essential in alkalinity. No, regular tap or bottled water is not going to cut it. Ionized or alkaline water is key to staying on track when living an alkaline lifestyle. It helps to get rid of the toxic acids in your system. Alkaline water is easier for your body to absorb, therefore it hydrates you more efficiently. It helps to oxygenate your blood and help to neutralize free radicals that are ravaging your body.

There are machines you can purchase for your home that will do it for you. We did that and I can honestly tell you it made a huge difference for us. You can also do as we do, and put lemon or lime juice straight into your fresh, filtered water. It has a very alkalizing effect on your system despite what many people think! No matter how you look at it, alkaline water is within your reach and a priceless addition to the alkaline lifestyle.

Note that just like in case of alkaline foods, alkaline water and alkaline drinks have got nothing to do with changing or raising your pH or even altering your blood pH. Alkaline drinks are simple, clean, toxin-free and preservatives free. Natural vitamins and minerals are also great. This is why we love infusing our water with some fresh fruits and herbs. Herbal, caffeine-free infusions are also alkaline in their design. They provide nutrients and have no caffeine.

We suggest you have a look at some basic Water Filter Pitchers. We got ours for only $30.We don't recommend bottled water, besides it may turn out to be quite expensive.

Start creating your fresh, fruit infused water today and keep hydrated. Try to drink more juices and smoothies.

If your goal is weight loss, detoxification and more energy, we recommend you juice: cucumbers, fennel, ginger, tomatoes, limes and lemons, spinach and other leafy greens + you may also add small pieces of other fruit to taste. Although we don't recommend juicing fruits high in sugar. It's better to have them as a snack or blend them and have them as smoothies.

Greens, greens, greens- they are the best, natural alkaline superfoods. You don't need to spend hundreds of dollars on some exotic superfoods and herbs from the other side of the world. Don't even worry about them. Focus on the abundance of fruits and veggies around you.

Talking about greens....

CHLOROPHYLL

One of the secrets to alkalinity that we have found is liquid chlorophyll. Yes, the same thing plants use for energy will help to energize you as well. Not to mention that it will also help to detoxify your body. You can get it by eating your vegetables, but why not add even more through your liquid intake as well?

You can find chlorophyll in concentrates. You simply mix in with your water and you are adding instant alkalinity to your system. It is available in powder form, liquid and super concentrated drops.

When you process chlorophyll, it actually increases the amount of red blood cells in the body. It also enables them to work more efficiently. It helps to restore our bodies' molecules and cells.

Chlorophyll is also:

- An anti-toxin. It will protect you from the pollutants from fungus-producing foods, meats, and pollution that we breathe.

- An anti-oxidant. Chlorophyll contains vitamin A, C, and E in large quantities making it a strong antioxidant. It prevents harmful inflammation.

- A detox for heavy metals. Chlorophyll attaches itself to heavy metals and allows your body to rid itself of them.

- A way to prevent candida. Chlorophyll helps your body to be resistant to candida and to be an environment where it cannot thrive.

- An avenue to get more magnesium. Chlorophyll contains a large amount of magnesium. It is a very alkalizing mineral. It helps our bodies to efficiently distribute enough oxygen to our cells. This enables us to build stronger bones and allows us to have maximum nerve function. It is very essential for every system in the body; all systems depend on magnesium.

Here is a mini chart that you can keep around that has some key substitutes for things you might miss from your normal diet. It makes it easier for us to not fall off the wagon!

-Replace Butter with Cold pressed oil (we love coconut oil)

-Replace Fruit in a can with Frozen or fresh fruit

-Replace Coffee with herbal Tea

-Replace Mayo with alkaline vegetable Hummus

-Replace Wheat flour with Almond flour

-Replace Peanuts with Almonds

-Replace Sugar with Stevia

-Replace Potatoes with Sweet Potatoes

-Replace White rice with Quinoa

-Replace Eggs with chia seed eggs (although we believe that organic eggs are good for you and can be eaten as a 20-30%part of your diet)

-Replace Yeast with lemon juice/baking soda

-Replace Regular Bread with Sprouted grain bread or wraps

Staying motivated is fueled by choices, as is anything in life. Here are a couple tips to help you make good alkaline choices.

- ✓ Always choose a meat substitute or poultry/fish over red fatty meat

- ✓ Drink hemp, almond or coconut milk over dairy

- ✓ Plan your meals centered around veggies-they should be the focus not the side dish

- ✓ If you cover your plate in greens you will not have room for the bad stuff

- ✓ Use cold-pressed oils over butter

- ✓ If eating out always order massive amount of salad with your main meal

- ✓ Always try to snack on fresh vegetables or fruits, no packaged snacks

Chapter 5 Paleo and Alkaline: The Best of Both Worlds

As a couple, James and I have always been concerned with health and wellness. We do not really consider anything a "diet." Eating well (or even poorly) is a lifestyle choice. In general I, Elena, was pretty healthy with my eating habits. I also preferred not to eat animals or their byproducts. This is not because I am an avid PETA supporter or anything, I just felt better as a whole when I was not consuming these foods. I had always eaten semi-vegan and enjoyed it. James, on the other hand, loves meat and eggs. He has been known to say that he might die without bacon. His favorite lifestyle change we made was Paleo. After delving into the world of alkalinity, we realized that we could probably have the best of both worlds. If you notice, many alkaline foods are paleo friendly, and vice-versa!

We started on this new paleo/alkaline adventure about a month ago. We have both lost even more weight using the two in conjunction. We seem to have more energy. The plateau we had both hit in regard to fat-loss has even been conquered.

There are many food lists available for each lifestyle. We just found the foods conducive to both lifestyles and started coming up with recipes. You can do the same! Who would not want to experience the benefits of these lifestyles? We want to share with you some of our recipes so that you can experience the benefit of combining paleo and alkaline eating as well!

Good fats have amino acids that are as essential to good health as alkalizing vegetables. Nuts and other vegetable proteins do not contain these fats.

Basically, this is how we eat: we eat 80% alkaline foods and 20% acidic foods (alkaline). The difference is, our twenty percent consists of meat (paleo).

Paleo+Alkaline is also great because you are able to detox. Strictly paleo diets do not focus much on detox. In this combination lifestyle you can add alkaline detox juices. This will help to detox your system, along with all of the vegetables you will be incorporating. Every paleo diet can benefit from an alkaline detox. By combining the two diets you can have your proverbial cake and eat it too!

Just make sure your 80% alkaline foods are paleo-acceptable (this is not hard). Make sure that you are devoting the other 20% to good fat filled, non-processed meats. We no longer waste our twenty percent on things that are not rich in good fats.

Here are a few recipes we have grown to love:

Alkaline Kale Salad with Lemon Salmon

- 8 c. chopped kale

- 2 c. diced red bell pepper (de-seeded)

- 2 tablespoons fresh mint (finely chopped)

- 4 tablespoons raw hemp seeds

- 2 tablespoons raw sunflower seeds

- 3 cloves minced garlic

- ¼ tsp cayenne

Dressing:

- ¼ c. evoo (cold pressed)

- 3 tablespoons lemon juice

- 2 tablespoons raw apple cider vinegar

- ¼ tablespoon fresh squeezed ginger

- Pinch sea salt

1. Put chopped and de-ribbed kale into a large mixing bowl.

2. Mix all ingredients for the dressing in another bowl.

3. Apply dressing to kale and mix with your hands.

4. Add all other ingredients and mix well.

5. Chill salad while cooking salmon.

Lemon Salmon

- 2 lb piece salmon

- 1 large sliced lemon

- 1 tablespoon capers

- Pepper to taste

- 1 tablespoon fresh thyme

- Oil to drizzle over

1. Put parchment paper on a cookie sheet.

2. Put salmon on the sheet, meat side up. Season with the pepper to your liking.

3. Put on capers and the put the sliced lemon, topping with thyme.

4. Do not preheat oven. Set it to 400 degrees when you put in the salmon.

5. Cook for 26 minutes and serve with Kale salad!

Alkaline Roast Veggies and Roast Chicken Drumsticks

- 1 cup sliced carrots

- 1 cup sliced parsnip

- 1 cup Brussels sprouts

- 1 large onion, chopped

- 1 cup dandelion greens

- Handful fresh basil

- Pinch sea salt and pepper

- 1 cup whole mushrooms

- 1 cup chopped and seeded bell pepper

- 4 Tablespoons evoo

- 1 tsp thyme

1. Preheat oven to 375 degrees.

2. Put vegetables on a greased sheet or pan. Season with spices and herbs, drizzling evoo immediately after. Bake for 45 minutes or until nicely browned. (Chicken will be cooking at the same time)

Roast Drumsticks

- 8 Drumsticks

- 1 teaspoon sea salt

- ½ teaspoon both garlic and onion powder

- 1 ½ tablespoon coconut oil

1. Combine all ingredients in a large bowl and brush over chicken in a 9x13 pan.

2. Bake with the vegetables for 45 min or until chicken reaches 165 degrees.

3. If you like it crispier like James, use tongs and flip over chicken and cook for an additional 6 minutes.

Serve with roasted veggies and enjoy!!

Grilled Veggies with Egg

- 8 mushrooms

- 2 large bunch asparagus

- 3 tablespoons evoo

- Salt and pepper to taste

- 3 eggs (poached)

Topping:

- ¼ c. evoo

- 2 tablespoons lemon juice

- 1 diced garlic clove

- ¼ tsp cayenne

- 1 tablespoon chopped parsley

1. Preheat the broiler to medium high (you can also barbeque but we like this for breakfast).

2. Coat veggies in oil and sprinkle with salt and pepper. Cook for 9 minutes under broiler or 3 minutes on each side on the barbeque.

3. Remove from heat and cover with foil.

4. Poach your eggs by putting approximately 4 inches of water in a saucepan.

5. Get the water hot enough to where it is almost boiling. Add 2 tsp. vinegar.

6. Work eggs in one at a time. Crack them into a cup and angle it slightly into the water, allowing egg to slide in. Use a spoon to keep whites near yolks.

7. Turn off burner and cover the sauce pan for about 3-4 min. Egg whites will look firm and white when ready. Remove with a slotted spoon.

8. Put dressing ingredients into bowl and whisk or stir with fork.

9. Plate veggies, top with eggs and then dressing.

10. Serve immediately and enjoy!

Alkaline Detox Juice

- Head of Celery

- Whole cucumber

- 4 Kale leaves

- 1 c. dandelion greens

- 1 Lemon (no peel)

- 1 tablespoon grated ginger

- ½ c. alfalfa sprouts

- 1 c. both parsley and cilantro

1. Juice all and enjoy!!!

Free Complimentary eBook

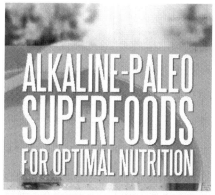

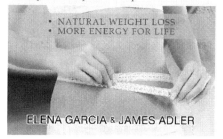

Grab your free copy now!

Download link:

www.bitly.com/alkapaleofree

Problems with your download?

Contact us: elenajamesbooks@gmail.com

Conclusion

Thank you again for downloading our book!

We hope we were able to help you understand the way that an alkaline lifestyle will completely change your body and mind, allowing you to get the most out of both. Our bodies function best when we nourish our body with alkaline nutrients. Altering your diet and embracing this lifestyle will allow you to live your life to the fullest.

Now that you know exactly how and what to do, do not waste another second in your toxic state. You deserve the best, and in order to achieve all of your goals in life you must be able to function efficiently: both mentally and physically.

Prevention is the best medicine, and keeping your body in an alkaline state is the best way to prevent disease. Why wait for disease to ravage the body before doing something about it? It is easier to prevent disease than to try and attack it.

We hope you will embrace this new lifestyle with open arms today. Learning about an alkaline lifestyle is the first step in becoming the best you that you can possibly be. We have given you the "how-tos," the "whys," and the tools to jump right in. You will not be sorry. The next step is just to do it.

We wish you the best on your journey to holistic health. It is our hope that we have helped to enlighten you as to the benefits of alkalinity.

Finally, if you enjoyed this book, please take the time to share your thoughts and post a review on Amazon. It would be greatly appreciated!

Thank you and good luck!

Elena and James
www.HolisticWellnessBooks.com

Similar Books by Elena and James

You will find them in your local Amazon store

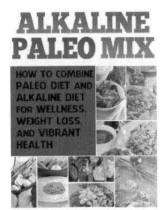 Kindle & Paperback

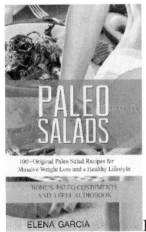 Kindle & Paperback

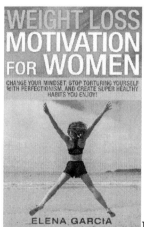

Kindle, Paperback & Audible

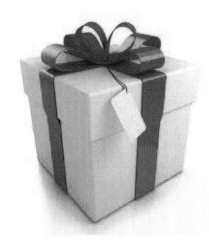

Don't forget to download your free gifts:

1. Free eBook:

   www.bitly.com/alkapaleofree

2. Printable charts:

   www.bitly.com/alkalinecharts

Printed in Poland
by Amazon Fulfillment
Poland Sp. z o.o., Wrocław